[TYPE THE COMPANY NAME]

Cortical bone has a complex hierarchical microstructure and is capable of self repair

Review

Rafis ismail

3/3/2014

Abstract

Bone's mechanical competence and its fragility in particular depend to a certain extent on the structure and microstructure of the cortical bone compartment. Beyond bone mineral density (BMD) and bone mineral content, a variety of other features of cortical bone contribute to whole bone's resistance to fracture. Structural properties of cortical bone most commonly employed as surrogate for its mechanical competence include thickness of the cortex, cortical cross-sectional area and area moment of inertia. But microstructural properties such as cortical porosity, crystallinity or the presence of microcracks also contribute to bone's mechanical competence. Microcracks in particular not only weaken the cortical bone tissue but also provide an effective mechanism for energy dissipation. Bone is a damageable, viscoelastic composite and most of all a living material capable of self-repair and thus exhibits a complex repertoire of mechanical properties. This review provides an overview of a variety of features of cortical bone known to provide mechanical competence and how these features may be applied for fracture risk prediction.

Contents

1.1 INTRODUCTION

Bone's mechanical competence and its fragility in particular depend to a certain extent on the structure and microstructure of the cortical bone compartment. Beyond bone mineral density (BMD) and bone mineral content, a variety of other features of cortical bone contribute to whole bone's resistance to fracture. Structural properties of cortical bone most commonly employed as surrogate for its mechanical competence include thickness of the cortex, cortical cross-sectional area and area moment of inertia. But microstructural properties such as cortical porosity, crystallinity or the presence of microcracks also contribute to bone's mechanical competence. Microcracks in particular not only weaken the cortical bone tissue but also provide an effective mechanism for energy dissipation. Bone is a damageable, viscoelastic composite and most of all a living material capable of self-repair and thus exhibits a complex repertoire of mechanical properties. This review provides an overview of a variety of features of cortical bone known to provide mechanical competence and how these features may be applied for fracture risk prediction.

1.2 STRUCTURAL PROPERTIES

From a mechanical perspective, it is quite obvious that the rigidity and strength of a structure is determined not only by the amount of material but even more importantly by the arrangement of the material in space. Geometrical measures such as bone size, cross-sectional area or area moment of inertia have frequently shown to predict up to 70–80% of whole bone strength. Biomechanical studies have evaluated the relative contributions of the different bone compartments and the geometric features to the mechanical strength of whole bone specimens. For the distal radius, the best predictors of fracture load are measures of cortical bone mass, cortical area and cortical width [1]. For the proximal femur cortical area, size of the femoral neck and area moment of inertia have been shown to be the strongest predictors of fracture load beyond BMD measurements [1, 2]. The combination of individual parameters in multiple regression models has provided further evidence that geometrical measurements considerably improve the prediction of bone strength [3]. Finally, computational models (finite element models) considering the entire arrangement of bone material in space, the local material properties and the anticipated direction of loading have provided the most accurate prediction of bone strength [4].

Retrospective studies confirmed the association of geometrical properties with the occurrence of fractures, mostly of fractures of the femoral neck [5]. Another predominant geometrical feature observed in femoral neck fractures is local thinning of cortical bone by endocortical resorption [6]. Bone geometry changes with age, adapting to a modified mechanical environment. Bone loss in the femoral neck is therefore lowest in those regions that bear the largest loads during normal gait, whereas cortical thickness is reduced in regions that are primarily loaded during falling. In the femoral shaft, a similar mechanism has been reported long ago [7]. In the distal forearm, the age-related adaptation is reflected in endosteal absorption together with periosteal apposition, increasing the area moment of inertia and thus preserving bone rigidity and strength [8]. Although this adaptive response has been observed in both women and men, it appears to be more effective in men.

1.3 MATERIAL PROPERTIES

Bone is a composite material containing about 70% mineral (hydroxyapatite), 22% proteins (type I collagen) and 8% water by weight. The material properties of cortical bone are determined by the quality and the spatial arrangement of these bone constituents. During everyday activity, bone has to withstand both compressive and tensile stresses and bending and torsional moments. Although the mineral constituent resists compression forces very effectively, it has a relatively poor ability to withstand tensile loads. In contrast, the tensile strength of bone results from the collagen fibrils arranged in lamellae. As forces and moments act not only from one direction, the orientation of the collagen fibrils varies between adjacent lamellae. Cortical bone is loaded mostly by bending moments, resulting in a high percentage of tensile strain. The structural quality therefore depends highly on the quality and orientation of its collagen fibrils. Furthermore, stiffness of cortical bone is predominantly associated with mineral content and bone density, whereas its toughness is strongly associated with the quality of the collagen matrix [9]. Although the mineral phase imparts strength and stiffness to bone tissue, with increasing mineralization, bone becomes brittle and requires less energy to fail. The collagen phase on the other hand provides toughness for cortical bone. If collagen denatures or its composition is altered, cortical bone toughness is reduced [10].

1.3.1 CRYSTAL

Besides structural properties and BMD, the mechanical properties of cortical bone depend on the size and distribution of mineral crystals [11]. Bone mineralization starts with multiple nucleations of crystals within the collagen fibrils. Crystal size increases by the addition of ions and by the aggregation of crystals, called 'secondary nucleation'. Factors affecting mineral crystal size are the collagen fibrils and other matrix proteins, as well as bone diseases, drugs, diet and age [12]. In young bone, a composition of recently formed small crystals and mature large crystals can be found. This mixture of small and large crystals may represent the optimal situation for good resistance to load. In ageing bone, the average crystal size increases. Bone becomes more brittle because of the greater number of large crystals and tends to fracture more easily. Deviation from the ideal composition is therefore considered to be associated with the deterioration of mechanical properties.

1.3.2 POROSITY

Haversian canals and resorption cavities in cortical bone produce a porous bone tissue with pore diameters ranging from a few up to several hundred micrometres (Figure 1). Morphometry and biomechanical testing have perceived strong correlations between intracortical porosity and cortical bone material properties. The number and size of the pores determine intracortical porosity, which accounts for about 70% of elastic modulus and 55% of yield stress (Figure 2) [13]. Local BMD measurements in cortical bone specimens have corroborated these findings [14]. Fracture toughness also decreases significantly with increasing porosity possibly by reducing the available area for the propagation of microcracks [15].

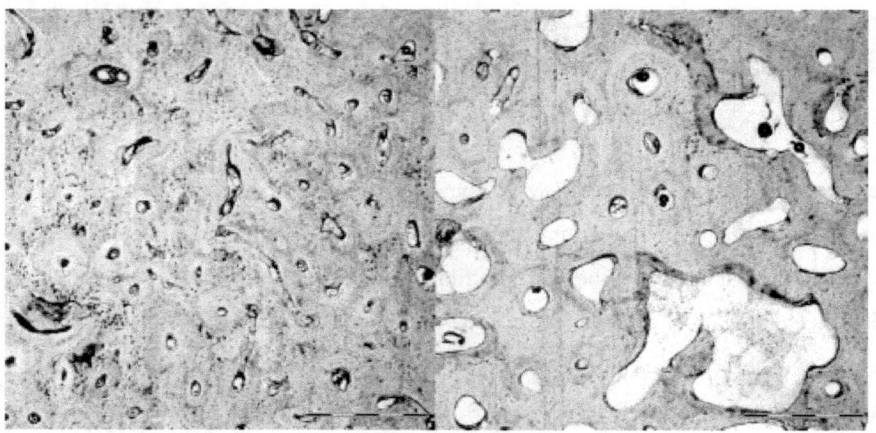

Fig. 1: Areas of dense (left) and porous (right) cortical bone from the femoral shaft of a 78-year-old woman. Light microscopic image at 25-fold magnification, Paragon staining.

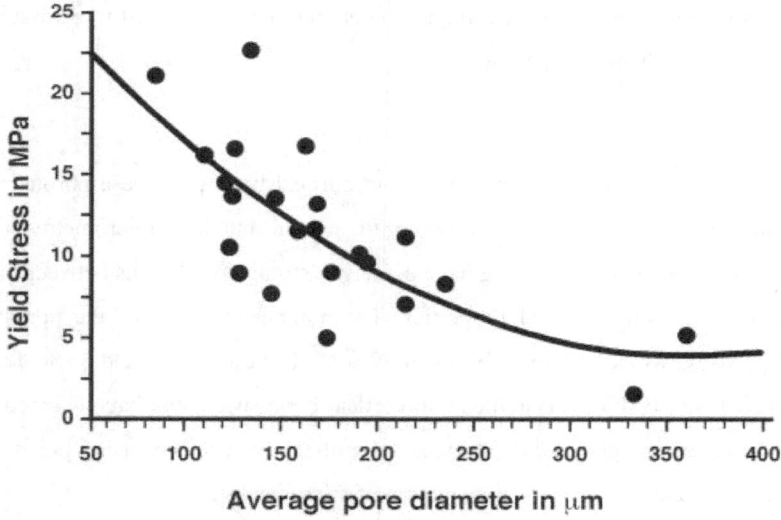

Fig. 2: Porosity of human cortical bone measured as average pore diameter is clearly related with decreasing material properties ($n = 23$, R2 = 0.54, $P<0.001$ [14]).

1.3.3 MICROCRACKS

Cortical bone is a composite material in which microcracks accumulate as a consequence of prolonged loading and result in bone fatigue. Microcracks are short splits in cortical bone tissue typically in the order of 30–100 μm in length with a 'linear' morphology and result from the disruption of intermolecular bonds (Figure 3) [16]. There may additionally be more diffuse matrix damages at various levels of the hierarchical sub lamellar architecture contributing to cortical bone's mechanical behavior [17]. The propagation of microcracks is frequently observed along cement lines because the osteonal cement lines have a lower resistance to crack propagation. Thus, the majority of microcracks are found between cement lines and the surrounding interstitial tissue. Microcracks occur during fatigue loading of cortical bone and are associated with a significant degradation of bone stiffness. Diffuse damage in particular coincides with yielding of bone. Microcracks occur through everyday activities, accumulate with age and are regularly found throughout the skeleton at load-bearing sites. Microcracks can also be induced during the loading event in a failure process of bone [18]. The generation of new micro cracks is a way of dissipating energy during a loading event by local formation of diffuse micro damage. The suppression of crack growth appears to be more important in preventing failure than the suppression of crack initiation [19]. Although microcracks formation is thought to be an effective way of energy dissipation, microcracks also impose adverse effects on the mechanical competence of bone. Stiffness and strength have been shown to decrease as the number of microdamages in bone increases [20]. It remains unclear, however, to what extent microdamage accumulation contributes to an increase in fracture risk.

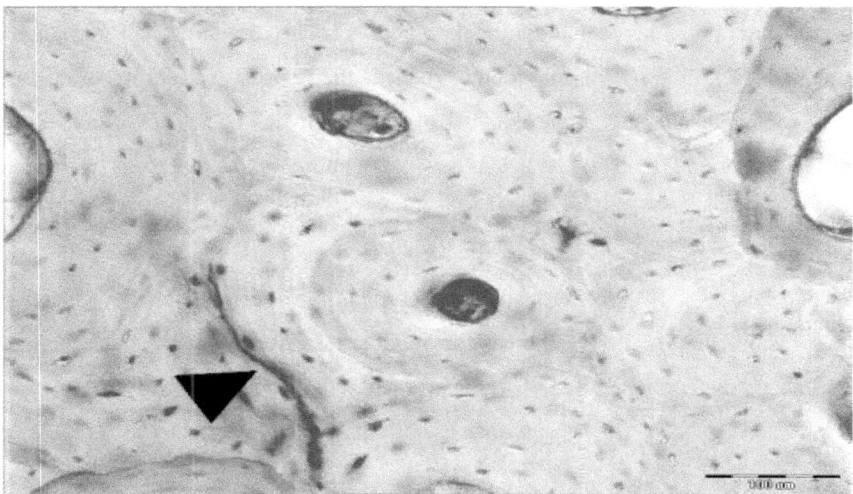

Fig.3: Microcracks (black arrow) in human cortical bone propagating partly along a cement line. Light microscopic image at 100-fold magnification, Paragon staining.

1.3.4 CHANGES WITH AGE

From a mechanical perspective, age-related degradation appears to be more pronounced for mechanical properties associated with tissue failure than for those associated with tissue stiffness [21]. Although energy absorption, fracture toughness and ultimate tensile strain show age-related changes of about 5–10% per decade, elastic module in tension or compression degrade by only about 2% per decade [22]. It appears, therefore, that the relationship between stiffness properties and failure properties changes with increasing tissue maturity. This is especially problematic because non-invasive image assessment measures mineral density, which is more closely related to stiffness properties than to failure strength or toughness.

Changes in bone's mechanical competence are explained by functional adaptation of bone structure and age-related deterioration of intrinsic mechanical properties. This deterioration is directly related to the bone remodeling process. Each osteonal remodeling event fails to replace all the bone previously removed and results in an increase in cortical bone porosity. The ratio of highly mineralized to new, less mineralized bone tissue is increased when bone remodeling is suppressed, resulting in an increase in the homogeneity of cortical bone tissue. A more homogenous tissue allows cracks to grow more easily and thus reduces the toughness of the composite material. An increased number of cement line interfaces may slow down crack propagation but may also serve as additional sources of crack initiation and may thus weaken cortical bone tissue. Furthermore, remodeling reduces the regional variability of collagen fiber orientation, leading to changes in mechanical properties. It has been shown that the collagen network itself experiences up to 50% loss in its capability to absorb energy during ageing probably because of an increase in the percentage of denatured collagen [23]. With increasing age, the degree of mineralization increases, which is reflected in an increase in mineral content of cortical bone tissue [24]. As microdamage in cortical bone accumulates with increasing age, there is a concomitant progressive increase in microcracks density [25]. After the age of 50, microcracks accumulate much more quickly in women than in men.

1.4 BONE MODELING

A particular feature of the bone is its ability to adapt its shape and size in response to mechanical loads. This mechanical adaptation is generated by a process known as modeling, in which bones are shaped or reshaped by the independent action of osteoblasts and osteoclasts. Modeling occurs vigorously not only during growth, but also, in the adult, in response to a mechanical load such as in tennis players in whom the radius of the playing arm has a thicker cortex and a larger external diameter than the contra lateral radius. Conversely, rapid bone loss may be induced by the unloading of the skeleton during bed rest or space flight [26].

Bone modeling differs from bone remodeling, because in this process bone formation is not coupled with prior bone resorption. The modeling process is less frequent than the remodeling one, but it does occur in normal subjects [27] and may be increased by some pathological states [28, 29].

1.5 BONE REMODELING

Bone remodeling is a lifelong process where in old bone is removed from the skeleton (a sub- process called bone resorption), and new bone is added (a sub-process called ossification or bone formation). Remodeling involves continuous removal of discrete packets of old bone, replacement of these packets with newly synthesized proteinaceous matrix, and subsequent mineralization of the matrix to form new bone [30, 31]. These processes also control the reshaping or replacement of bone during growth and following injuries like fractures but also microdamage (prevents accumulation of bone microdamage through replacement of old bone with the new one) [32] which occurs during normal activity. Remodeling responds also to functional demands of the mechanical loading. As a result, bone is added where needed and removed where it is not required. This process is essential in the maintenance of bone strength and mineral homeostasis. The skeleton is a metabolically active organ that undergoes continuous remodeling throughout life. This remodeling is necessary both to maintain the structural integrity of the skeleton and to subserve its metabolic functions as a storehouse of calcium and phosphorus.

Normal bone remodeling cycle requires that the process of bone resorption and bone formation take place in a coordinated fashion, which in turn depends on the orderly development and activation of osteoclasts and osteoblasts, respectively. This property of bone, which constantly resorbs the old bone and forms new bone, makes the bone a very dynamic tissue that permits the maintenance of bone tissue, the repair of damaged tissue, and the homeostasis of the phosphocalcic metabolism. The bone remodeling cycle involves a series of highly regulated steps that depend on the interactions of two cell lineages, the mesenchymal osteoblastic lineage and the hematopoietic osteoblastic lineage [31]. The balance between bone resorption and bone deposition is determined by the activities of these two principle cell types, namely, osteoclasts and osteoblasts. Osteoblasts and osteoclasts, coupled together via paracrine cell signaling, are referred to as bone remodeling units.

In the young skeleton, the amount of resorbed bone is proportional to the newly formed. For this reason, it is referred to as a balanced process, linked in both space and time under normal conditions. The average lifespan of each remodeled unit in humans is 2–8 months, the greater part of this time being taken up by bone formation. Bone remodeling occurs throughout life, but only up to the third decade is the balance positive. It is precisely in the third decade when the bone mass is at its maximum, and this is maintained with small variations until the age of 50. From then on, resorption predominates and the bone mass begins to decrease. Bone remodeling increases in premenopausal and early postmenopausal women and then slows with further aging but continues at a faster rate than in premenopausal women.

Although cortical bone makes up 75 % of the total volume, the metabolic rate is ten times higher in trabecular bone, since the surface area-to-volume ratio is much greater (trabecular bone surface representing 60 % of the total). Therefore, approximately 5–10 % of total bone is renewed per year.

Osteoclasts are endowed with highly active ion channels in the cell membrane that pump protons into the extracellular space, thus lowering the pH in their own microenvironment. This drop in pH dissolves the bone mineral [33].

The bone remodeling cycle involves a complex series of sequential steps (coupling of bone formation and bone resorption). Bone balance is the difference between the old bone resorbed and new bone formed. Periosteal bone balance is mildly positive, whereas endosteal and trabecular bone balances are mildly negative, leading to cortical and trabecular thinning with aging. These relative changes occur with endosteal resorption outstripping periosteal formation.

The main recognized functions of bone remodeling include preservation of bone mechanical strength by replacing older, microdamaged bone with newer, healthier bone and calcium and phosphate homeostasis. The relatively low adult cortical bone turnover rate of 2–3 %/year is adequate to maintain biomechanical strength of bone. The rate of trabecular bone turnover is higher, more than required for maintenance of mechanical strength, indicating that trabecular bone turnover is more important for mineral metabolism. Increased demand for calcium or phosphorus may require increased bone remodeling units.

1.6 MEDIATORS OF REMODELING

1.6.1 OSTEOCLASTS

Osteoclasts are the only cells that are known to be capable of resorbing bone. They are typically multinucleated. Osteoclasts are derived from mononuclear precursor cells of the monocyte-macrophage lineage (hematopoietic stem cells that give rise to monocytes and macrophages). [34] Mononuclear monocyte-macrophage precursor cells have been identified in various tissues, but bone marrow monocyte-macrophage precursor cells are thought to give rise to most osteoclasts.

1.6.2 OSTEOBLASTS

Osteoblasts can be stimulated to increase bone mass through increased secretion of osteoid and by inhibiting the ability of osteoclasts to break down osseous tissue. Bone building through increased formation of osteoid is stimulated by the secretion of growth hormone by the pituitary, the thyroid hormone and the sex hormones (estrogens and androgens).

1.6.3 RANK

The cell surface receptor called RANK (for receptor activator of NFkB) prods osteoclasts precursor cells to develop into fully differentiated osteoclasts when RANK is activated by its cognate partner RANK ligand (RANKL). RANKL belongs to the TNF super family and is critical for osteoclasts formation. It is one of the key signaling molecules that facilitate cross talk between the osteoblasts and osteoclasts and help coordinate bone remodeling. RANKL and macrophage CSF (M-CSF) are two cytokines that are critical for osteoclasts formation. Both RANKL and M-CSF are produced mainly by marrow stromal cells and osteoblasts in membrane-bound and soluble forms, and osteoclastogenesis requires the presence of stromal cells and osteoblasts in bone marrow [35, 36]. Osteoprotegerin is another protein released by osteoblasts that acts as a decoy to prevent RANK and RANKL from coming in contact [37, 34, 38, 39, 40, 41]. Osteoblast precursors express a molecule called TRANCE, or osteoclasts differentiation factor, which can activate cells of the osteoclasts lineage by interacting with a receptor called RANK [42, 41].

1.6.4 OSTEOPROTEGERIN

Osteoprotegerin (OPG), also known as osteoclasts inhibiting factor (OCIF) or osteoclasts binding factor (OBF), is a key factor inhibiting the differentiation and activation of osteoclasts, and is, therefore, essential for bone resorption. Osteoprotegerin is a dimeric glycoprotein belonging to the TNF receptor family. Osteoprotegerin inhibits the binding of RANK to RANKL and thus inhibits the recruitment, proliferation, and activation of osteoclasts. Abnormalities in the balance of OPGL/RANK/OPG system lead to the increased bone resorption that underlies the bone damage of postmenopausal osteoporosis, Paget's disease, bone loss in metastatic cancers, and rheumatoid arthritis. Bone resorption depends on osteoclasts secretion of hydrogen ions and cathepsin K enzyme. H+ ions acidify the resorption compartment beneath osteoclasts to dissolve the mineral component of bone matrix, whereas cathepsin K digests the proteinaceous matrix, which is mostly composed of type I collagen [34].

Osteoclasts bind to bone matrix via integrin receptors in the osteoclasts membrane linking to bone matrix peptides. They digest the organic matrix, resulting in formation of saucer-shaped Howship's lacunae on the surface of trabecular bone and Haversian canals in cortical bone. The resorption is completed by mononuclear cells after the multinucleated osteoclasts undergo apoptosis [43, 44, 45, 46]. The boundary between the old and new bone is distinguished in a hematoxylin and eosin section by a blue (basophilic) line called a cement line or reversal line.

1.6.5 PARACRINE CELL SIGNALING

At various stages throughout this process of remodeling, the precursors, osteoclasts, and osteoblasts communicate with each other through the release of various "signaling" molecules.

Osteoclasts are apparently activated by "signals" from osteoblasts. For example, osteoblasts have receptors for PTH, whereas osteoclasts do not, and PTH-induced osteoclastic bone resorption is said not to occur in the absence of osteoblasts. The action of osteoblasts and osteoclasts is controlled by a number of chemical factors which either promote or inhibit the activity of the bone remodeling cells, controlling the rate at which bone is made, destroyed, or changed in shape. The cells also use paracrine signaling to control the activity of each other.

1.7 REMODELING PHASES

Bone remodeling can be divided into the following six phases (Fig.4) namely, quiescent, activation, resorption, reversal, formation, and mineralization. Activation precedes resorption which precedes reversal, with mineralization as the last step These occur at remodeling sites which are distributed randomly but also are targeted to areas that require repair [47, 30, 48].

1. **Quiescent Phase.** It is the state/phase of the bone when at rest. The factors that initiate the remodeling process remain unknown.
2. **Activation Phase.** The first phenomenon that occurs is the activation of the bone surface prior to resorption, through the retraction of the bone lining cells (elongated mature osteoblasts existing on the endosteal surface) and the digestion of the endosteal membrane by collagenase action. The initial "activation" stage involves recruitment and activation of mononuclear monocyte-macrophage osteoclasts precursors from the circulation [49, 50], resulting in interaction of osteoclasts and osteoblasts precursor cells. This leads to the differentiation, migration, and fusion of the large multinucleated osteoclasts. These cells attach to the mineralized bone surface and initiate resorption by the secretion of hydrogen ions and lysosomal enzymes, particularly cathepsin K, which can degrade all the components of bone matrix, including collagen, at low pH.
3. **Resorption Phase** (Fig5). The osteoclasts then begin to dissolve the mineral matrix and decompose the osteoid matrix. This process is completed by the macrophages and permits the release of the growth factors contained within the matrix, fundamentally transforming growth factor- b (TGF- b), platelet-derived growth factor (PDGF), and insulin-like growth factor I and II (IGF- I and II). Osteoclastic resorption produces irregular scalloped cavities on the trabecular bone surface, called Howship's lacunae, or cylincrical Haversian canals in cortical

bone. Osteoclast-mediated bone resorption takes only approximately 2–4 weeks during each remodeling cycle.

4. **Reversal Phase**. During the reversal phase, bone resorption transitions to bone formation. At the completion of bone resorption, resorption cavities contain a variety of mononuclear cells, including monocytes, osteocytes released from bone matrix, and preosteoblasts, recruited to begin new bone formation. The coupling signals linking the end of bone resorption to the beginning of bone formation are as yet unknown, but proposed coupling signal candidates include bone matrix-derived factors such as TGF-/3, IGF-1, IGF-2, bone morphogenetic proteins, PDGF, or fibroblast growth factor [51, 52, 53].

5. **Formation Phase**. Once osteoclasts have resorbed a cavity of bone, they detach from the bone surface and are replaced by cells of the osteoblasts lineage which in turn initiate bone formation. The preosteoblasts grouping phenomenon is produced and attracted by the growth factors liberated from the matrix which act as chemotactics and in addition stimulate their proliferation [54]. The preosteoblasts synthesize a cementing substance upon which the new tissue is attached and express bone morphogenic proteins (BMP) responsible for differentiation. A few days later, the already differentiated osteoblasts synthesize the osteoid matrix which fills the (resorption cavity) perforated areas [54]. The remaining osteoblasts continue to synthesize bone until they eventually stop and transform to quiescent lining cells that completely cover the newly formed bone surface and connect with the osteocytes in the bone matrix through a network of canaliculi.

6. **Mineralization Phase.** The process begins 30 days after deposition of the osteoid, ending at 90 days in the trabecular and at 130 days in the cortical bone. The quiescent or "at rest" phase then begins again. When the cycle is completed, the amount of bone formed should equal the amount of bone resorbed.

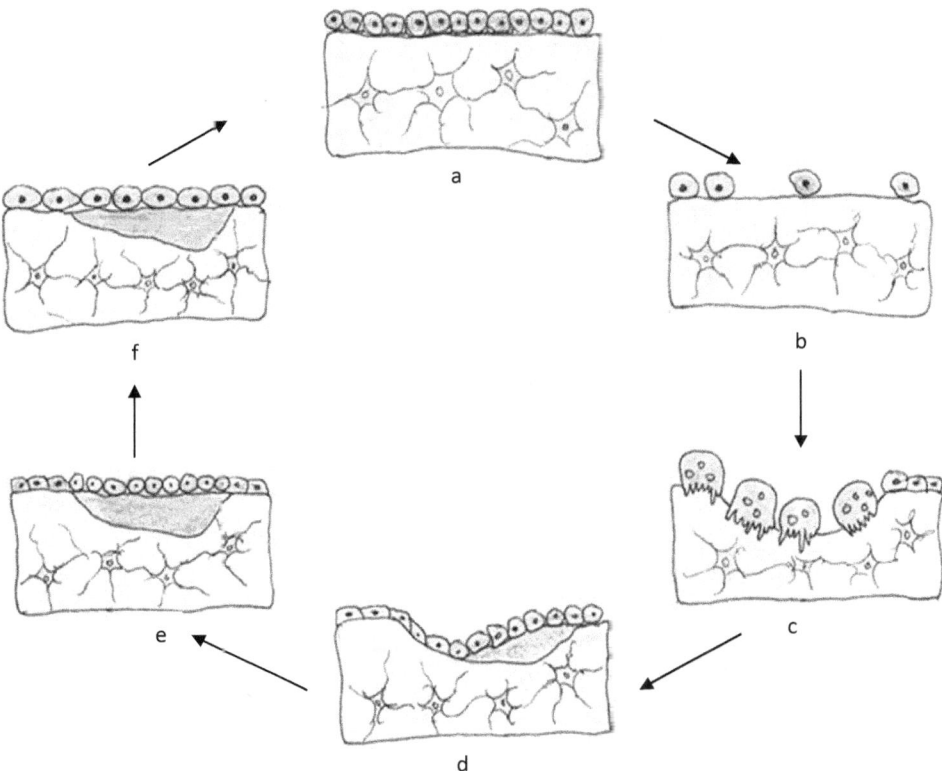

Fig.4: Phases of bone remodeling: (**a**) quiescent phase where flat bone lining cells are seen lining theendosteal membrane. (**b**) showing activation phase characterized by cell retraction with resultant membrane resorption. (**c**) shows activated osteoclasts resorbing the underlying bone. (**d**) shows formation phase where the osteoclasts are replaced by osteoblasts with underlying new osteoid matrix. (**e**) shows mineralization of osteoid matrix. (**f**) shows formation of bone structure unit with progression to quiescent phase.

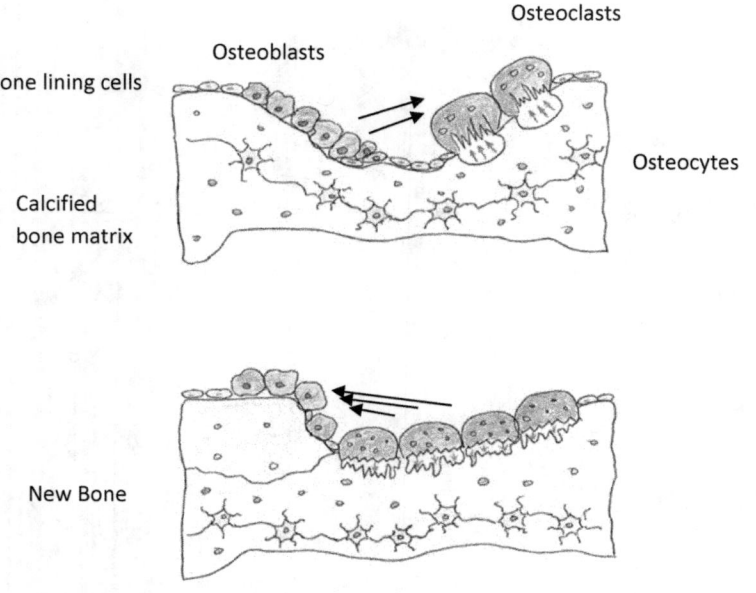

Fig. 5: To show normal bone remodeling (**a**) vs. defective resorption (**b**) seen in disease states

1.8 Regulatory Factors in Bone Remodeling

The balance between bone resorption and formation is influenced by such interrelated factors as genetic, mechanical, vascular, nutritional, hormonal, and local.

1.8.1 Systemic Regulation of Bone Remodeling

1. **Genetic factors** These are important in determining the maximum bone mass, since between 60 and 80 % of this bone mass is genetically determined. Thus, Negroes have a greater bone mass than Whites, who in turn have a higher mass than Asians. Bone mass is a characteristic transmitted from parents to children, which is why daughters of mothers with osteoporosis are more predisposed to having this condition themselves [55, 56].

2. **Mechanical Factors** Remodeling is regulated by mechanical loading, allowing bone to adapt its structure in response to the mechanical demands. Physical activity is essential for the correct development of bone. It is believed that muscular action transmits tension to the bone, which is detected by the osteocytes network within the osseous fluid. On the other hand, the

absence of muscular activity, rest, or weightlessness has an adverse effect on bone, accelerating resorption. It is well-known that trabeculae tend to align with maximum stresses in many bones. Mechanical stress improves bone strength by influencing collagen alignment as new bone is being formed. Cortical bone tissue located in regions subject to predominantly tensile stresses has a higher percentage of collagen fibers aligned along the bone long axis. In regions of predominant compressive stresses, fibers are more likely to be aligned transverse to the long axis.

3. **Vascular / Nerve Factors** Vascularization is fundamental for normal bone development, supplying blood cells, oxygen, minerals, ions, glucose, hormones, and growth factors. Vascularization constitutes the first phase in ossification: the blood vessels invade the cartilage and later produce resorption via the osteoclasts originating from the nearby vessels. In the same way, vascular neoformation is the first event in the repair of fractures or bone regeneration [57]. Innervaion is necessary for normal bone physiology. The bone is innervated by the autonomous nervous system and by sensorial nerve fibers. Autonomous fibers have been found in periosteum, endosteum, and cortical bone and associated with the blood vessels of the Volkmann conduit, and likewise neuropeptides and their receptors in bone [58]. Examples of the importance of innervations in bone physiology are found in osteopenia and the bone fragility present in patients with neurological disorders, and also in the decreased bone density in de-nerved mandibles.

4. **Nutritional Factors** A minimum amount of calcium is needed for mineralization, which the majority of authors put at 1,200 mg/day to the age of 25, not less than 1 g/day from 25 to 45, and following menopause should be at least 1,500 mg/day. Likewise, it is known that toxic habits such as smoking, caffeine, alcohol, and excess salt constitute risk factors for osteopenia.

5. **Hormonal Factors Normal** development of the skeleton is conditioned by the correct functioning of the endocrine system. The most important hormones in bone remodeling are:

(a) **Thyroid Hormones.** Thyroid hormones can also stimulate bone resorption and formation (possess two opposing actions on bone) and are critical for maintenance of normal bone remodeling [59]. In the first place, they stimulate the synthesis of the osteoid matrix by the osteoblasts and its mineralization, favoring the synthesis of IGF-I. For this reason, in congenital hypothyroidism (cretinism), short stature is produced by the alteration in bone formation. In the second place, a contrary effect is produced, stimulating resorption with the increase in number and function of the osteoclasts. The clinical manifestation of this effect is the appearance of bone loss in hyperthyroidism. (b) **Parathyroid Hormone (PTH).** It controls the homeostasis of calcium by direct action on the bone and the kidneys and indirectly on the intestine. It is produced by the parathyroid glands in response to hypocalcaemia. Continual supply of PTH would stimulate bone resorption through the synthesis of a factor favoring osteoclastogenesis (RANKL) on the part of the osteoblastic cells, while at intermittent doses it would stimulate the formation of bone, associated with an increase of the above-mentioned growth factors and with a decrease in the apoptosis of the osteoblasts. PTH regulates serum calcium concentration. It is a potent stimulator of bone resorption and has biphasic effects on bone formation. There is an acute inhibition of collagen synthesis with high concentrations of PTH, but prolonged intermittent administration of this hormone produces increased bone formation, a property for which it is being explored clinically as an anabolic agent [60]. Plasma PTH tends to increase with age, and this may produce an increase in bone turnover and a loss of bone mass, particularly of cortical bone. (c) **Calcitonin.** Produced by the parafollicular C cells of the thyroid, it is an inhibitor of bone resorption, reducing the number and activity of the osteoclasts. However, this is a transitory action, since the osteoclasts seem to become "impermeable" to calcitonin within a few days. (d) **1, 25(OH) 2Vitamin D3or Calcitriol.** A steroid hormone, by favoring the intestinal absorption of calcium and phosphate, favors bone mineralization. It is necessary for normal growth of the skeleton. Some authors believe it may be produced by lymphocytic or monocytic bone cells, playing an important role as a local regulator of osteoclasts differentiation [61]. (e) **Androgens.** Androgens have an anabolic effect on bone through the stimulation of the osteoblasts receptors. Likewise, they act as mediators of the growth hormone in puberty. While androgen deficiency is associated with lower bone density, the administration of testosterone in young people before the closure of the epiphyses increases bone mass. In the same way, women with an excess of androgens present higher bone densities. Androgens increase cortical bone size via stimulation of both longitudinal and radial growth. First, androgens, like estrogens, have a biphasic effect on endochondral bone formation: at the start of puberty, sex steroids stimulate endochondral bone formation, whereas they induce epiphyseal closure at the end of puberty. This effect of androgens may be important because bone strength in males seems to be determined by relatively higher periosteal bone formation and, therefore, greater bone dimensions, relative to muscle mass at older age. Androgens protect men against osteoporosis via maintenance of cancellous bone mass and expansion of cortical bone. (f) **Estrogens.** Estrogens are essential for the closure of the growth plates and have an important role in the development of the skeleton. Estrogens have a dual effect on bone metabolism: on the one hand, they favor bone formation, increasing the number and function of the osteoblasts, and on the other, they reduce resorption. Estrogen receptors have been described in human osteoblasts, osteocytes, and osteoclasts. Recent investigations have found that estrogens can increase the levels of osteoprotegerin (OPG), a protein produced by osteoblasts that inhibits resorption, so they may play an important role in the regulation of osteoclastogenesis [62]. Alternatively, estrogen may inhibit local factors that impair bone formation or enhance local factors that stimulate bone formation. For this reason, estrogen deficiency during menopause constitutes the most important pathogenic factor in bone loss associated with osteoporosis. Loss of estrogens or androgens increases the rate of bone remodeling by removing restraining effects on osteoblastogenesis and osteoclastogenesis and also causes a focal imbalance between resorption and formation by prolonging the lifespan of osteoclasts and shortening the lifespan of osteoblasts. (g) **Progesterone.** Progesterone also has an anabolic effect on bone, either directly, through the osteoblasts which possess hormone receptors, or indirectly, through competition for the osteoblastic receptors of the glucocorticoids. (h) **Insulin.** Insulin stimulates matrix synthesis both directly and indirectly, increasing the hepatic synthesis of IGF-I (insulin-like growth factor). (i) **Glucocorticoids.** Glucocorticoids are necessary for bone cell differentiation during development, but their greatest postnatal effect is to inhibit bone formation (at high doses, they have a catabolic effect on bone), since they inhibit the synthesis of IGF-I by the osteoblasts and directly suppress BMP-2, critical factors in osteoblasto genesis. This is the major pathogenetic mechanism in glucocorticoids-induced osteoporosis. Indirect effects of glucocorticoids on calcium absorption and sex hormone production may, however, increase bone resorption [63, 64]. (j) **Growth Hormone**. Growth hormone acts both directly and indirectly on bone. Growth hormone acts directly on the osteoblasts with hormone receptors, stimulating their activity, thus increasing the synthesis of collagen, osteocalcin, and alkaline phosphate. The indirect action is produced through an increase in synthesis of IGF-I and II by the osteoblasts. These factors stimulate the proliferation and differentiation of the osteoblasts, increasing their number and function [65, 66]. Thus, the hormones that regulate bone metabolism are as follows:

- Decrease bone resorption
  - Calcitonin
  - Estrogens
- Increase bone resorption
  - PTH/PTHrP
  - Glucocorticoids
  - Thyroid hormones
  - High-dose vitamin D
- Increase bone formation
  - Growth hormone
  - Vitamin D metabolites
  - Androgens –Insulin
  - Low-dose PTH/PTHrP
  - Progestogens
- Decrease bone formation
  - Glucocorticoids

REFERENCES

1. Augat P, Reeb H, Claes L. Prediction of fracture load at different skeletal sites by geometrical properties of the cortical shell. J Bone Miner Res 1996; 11: 1356–63.
2. Lochmuller EM, Groll O, Kuhn V, Eckstein F. Mechanical strength of the proximal femur as predicted from geometric and densitometric bone properties at the lower limb versus the distal radius. Bone 2002; 30: 207–16.
3. Lang TF, Keyak JH, Heitz MW et al. Volumetric quantitative computed tomography of the proximal femur: precision and relation to bone strength. Bone 1997; 21: 101–8.
4. Keyak JH, Falkinstein Y. Comparison of in situ and in vitro CT scan-based finite element model predictions of proximal femoral fracture load. Med Eng Phys 2003; 25: 781–7.
5. Gnudi S, Ripamonti C, Lisi L, Fini M, Giardino R, Giavaresi G. Proximal femur geometry to detect and distinguish femoral neck fractures from trochanteric fractures in postmenopausal women. Osteoporos Int 2002; 13: 69–73.
6. Crabtree N, Loveridge N, Parker M et al. Intracapsular hip fracture and the region-specific loss of cortical bone: analysis by peripheral quantitative computed tomography. J Bone Miner Res 2001; 16: 1318–28.
7. Martin RB, Atkinson PJ. Age and sex-related changes in the structure and strength of the human femoral shaft. J Biomech 1977; 10: 223–31.
8. Bouxsein ML, Myburgh KH, van der Meulen MC, Lindenberger E, Marcus R. Age-related differences in crosssectional geometry of the forearm bones in healthy women. Calcif Tissue Int 1994; 54: 113–8.
9. Zioupos P, Currey JD. Changes in the stiffness, strength, and toughness of human cortical bone with age. Bone 1998; 22: 57–66.
10. Zioupos P, Currey JD, Hamer AJ. The role of collagen in the declining mechanical properties of aging human cortical bone. J Biomed Mater Res 1999; 45: 108–16.
11. Martin B. Aging and strength of bone as a structural material. Calcif Tissue Int 1993; 53 (Suppl. 1): S34–9; discussion S39–40.
12. Boskey A. Bone mineral crystal size. Osteoporos Int 2003; 14 (Suppl. 5): 16–21.
13. Dong XN, Guo XE. The dependence of transversely isotropic elasticity of human femoral cortical bone on porosity. J Biomech 2004; 37: 1281–7.
14. Wachter NJ, Krischak GD, Mentzel M et al. Correlation of bone mineral density with strength and microstructural parameters of cortical bone in vitro. Bone 2002; 31: 90–5.
15. Yeni YN, Brown CU, Wang Z, Norman TL. The influence of bone morphology on fracture toughness of the human femur and tibia. Bone 1997; 21: 453–9.
16. Burr DB, Martin RB, Schaffler MB, Radin EL. Bone remodeling in response to in vivo fatigue microdamage. J Biomech 1985; 18: 189–200.
17. Schaffler MB. Bone fatigue and remodelling in the development of stress fractures. In: Burr DB, Milgrom C, eds. Musculoskeletal Fatigue and Stress Fractures. Boca Raton: CRC Press, 2001; 161–82.
18. Wang X, Puram S. The toughness of cortical bone and its relationship with age. Ann Biomed Eng 2004; 32: 123–35.
19. Burr D. Microdamage and bone strength. Osteoporos Int 2003; Suppl 5: 67–72.
20. Zioupos P. Accumulation of in-vivo fatigue microdamage and its relation to biomechanical properties in ageing human cortical bone. J Microsc 2001; 201: 270–8.
21. Jepsen KJ. The aging cortex: to crack or not to crack. Osteoporos Int 2003; 14 (Suppl. 5): 57–66.

22. Burstein AH, Reilly DT, Martens M. Aging of bone tissue: mechanical properties. J Bone Joint Surg Am 1976; 58: 82–6.
23. Wang X, Bank RA, TeKoppele JM, Agrawal CM. The role of collagen in determining bone mechanical properties. J Orthop Res 2001; 19: 1021–6.
24. Currey JD, Brear K, Zioupos P. The effects of ageing and changes in mineral content in degrading the toughness of human femora. J Biomech 1996; 29: 257–60.
25. Schaffler MB, Choi K, Milgrom C. Aging and matrix microdamage accumulation in human compact bone. Bone 1995; 17: 521–5.
26. Haapasalo H, Kontulainen S, Sievanen H, Kannus P, Jarvinen M, Vuori I. Exercise-induced bone gain is due to enlargement in bone size without a change in volumetric bone density: a peripheral quantitative computed tomography study of the upper arms of male tennis players. Bone 2000; 27:351-7.
27. Kobayashi S, Takahashi HE, Ito A, et al. Trabecular minimodeling in human iliac bone. Bone 2003; 32:163-9.
28. Ubara Y, Fushimi T, Tagami T, et al. Histomorphometric features of bone in patients with primary and secondary hypoparathyroidism. Kidney Int 2003; 63:1809-16.
29. Ubara Y, Tagami T, Nakanishi S, et al. Significance of mini-modeling in dialysis patients with adynamic bones disease. Kidney Int 2005; 68:833-9.
30. Fernández-Tresguerres-Hernández-Gil I, Alobera-Gracia MA, del Canto-Pingarrón M et al (2006) Physiological bases of bone regeneration II. The remodeling process. Med Oral Patol Oral Cir Bucal 11:E151–E157
31. Fraher L (1993) Biochemical markers of bone turnover. Clin Biochem 26:431–432
32. Turner CH (1998) Three rules for bone adaptation to mechanical stimuli. Bone 23:339–409
33. Blair HC, Teitebaum SL, Ghiselli R et al (1989) Osteoclastic bone resorption by a polarized vacuolar proton pump. Science 245:855–857
34. Boyle WJ, Simonet WS, Lacey DL (2003) Osteoclast differentiation and activation. Nature 423:337–342
35. Teitelbaum SL, Ross FP (2003) Genetic regulation of osteoclast development and function. Nat Rev Genet 4:638–649
36. Cohen MM Jr (2006) The new bone biology: pathologic, molecular, clinical correlates. Am J Med Genet A 140:2646–2706
37. Asagiri M, Takayanagi H (2007) The molecular understanding of osteoclast differentiation. Bone 40:251–264
38. Lacey DL, Timms E, Tan HL et al (1998) Osteoprotegerin ligand is a cytokine that regulates osteoclast differentiation and activation. Cell 93:165–176
39. Suda T, Takahashi N, Udagawa N et al (1999) Modulation of osteoclast differentiation and function by the new members of the tumor necrosis factor receptor and ligand families. Endocr Rev 20:345–357
40. Theill LE, Boyle WJ, Penninger JM (2002) RANK-L and RANK: T cells, bone loss, and mammalian evolution. Annu Rev Immunol 20:795–823
41. Yasuda H, Shima N, Nakagawa N et al (1998) Osteoclast differentiation factor is a ligand for osteoprotegerin/osteoclastogenesis-inhibitory factor and is identical to TRANCE/RANKL. Proc Natl Acad Sci USA 95:3597–3602

42. Horwood NJ, Elliott J, Martin TJ et al (1998) Osteotropic agents regulate the expression of osteoclast differentiation factor and osteoprotegerin in osteoblastic stromal cells. Endocrinology 139:4743–4746

43. Eriksen EF (1986) Normal and pathological remodeling of human trabecular bone: three dimensional reconstruction of the remodeling sequence in normals and in metabolic bone disease. Endocr Rev 7:379–408

44. Reddy SV (2004) Regulatory mechanisms operative in osteoclasts. Crit Rev Eukaryot Gene Expr 14:255–270

45. Teitelbaum SL, Abu-Amer Y, Ross FP (1995) Molecular mechanisms of bone resorption. J Cell Biochem 59:1–10

46. Vaananen HK, Zhao H, Mulari M et al (2000) The cell biology of osteoclast function. J Cell Sci 113:377–381

47. Burr DB (2002) Targeted and nontargeted remodeling. Bone 30:2–4

48. Parfitt AM (2002) Targeted and nontargeted bone remodeling: relationship to basic multicellular unit origination and progression. Bone 30:5–7

49. Bruzzaniti A, Baron R (2007) Molecular regulation of osteoclast activity. Rev Endocr Metab Disord 7: 123–139

50. Roodman GD, Kurihara N, Ohsaki Y et al (1992) Interleukin-6: a potential autocrine/paracrine agent in Paget's disease of bone. J Clin Invest 89:46–52

51. Bonewald LF, Mundy GR (1990) Role of transforming growth factor beta in bone remodeling. Clin Orthop Relat Res 2S:35–40

52. Hock JM, Centrella M, Canalis E et al (2004) Insulin-like growth factor I (IGF-I) has independent effects on bone matrix formation and cell replication. Endocrinology 122:254–260

53. Locklin RM, Oreffo RO, Trif fi tt JT et al (1999) Effects of TGFbeta and bFGF on the differentiation of human bone marrow stromal fi broblasts. Cell Biol Int 23:185–194

54. Lind M, Deleuran B, Thestrup-Pedersen K et al (1995) Chemotaxis of human osteoblasts. Effects of osteotropic growth factors. APMIS 103:140–146

55. Grant SFA, Ralston SH (1997) Genes and osteoporosis. Endocrinology 8:232–239

56. Pocock NA, Eisman JA, Hopper JL et al (1987) Genetic determinants of bone mass in adults: a twin study. J Clin Invest 80:706–710

57. Trueta J (1963) The role of blood vessels in osteogenesis. J Bone Joint Surg Br 45:402

58. Wheeless CR. http://www.wheelessonline.com/ortho/bone_remodeling. Accessed 20 Apr 2011

59. Kawaguchi H, Pilbeam CC, Raisz LG (1994) Anabolic effects of 3,3',5- triiodothyronine and triiodothyroacetic acid in cultured neonatal mouse parietal bones. Endocrinology 135:971–976

60. Dempster DW, Cosman F, Parisien M et al (1993) Anabolic actions of parathyroid hormone on bone. Endocr Rev 14:690–709

61. Raisz LG (1993) Bone cell biology: new approaches and unanswered questions. J Bone Miner Res 8:457–465

62. Hofbauer LC, Khosla S, Dunstan CR et al (1999) Estrogen stimulates gene expression and protein production of osteoprotegerin in human osteoblastic cells. Endocrinology 140:4367–4370

63. Lukert BP, Kream BE (1996) Clinical and basic aspects of glucocorticoid action in bone. In: Bilezikian JP, Raisz LG, Rodan GA (eds) Principles of bone biology. Academic, San Diego, pp 533–548
64. Manolagas SC (2000) Birth and death of bone cells: basic regulatory mechanisms and implications for the pathogenesis and treatment of osteoporosis. Endocr Rev 21:115–137
65. Harvey S, Hull KL (1998) Growth hormone: a paracrine growth factor? Endocrine 7:267–279
66. Rosen CJ, Donahue LR (1998) Insulin-like growth factors and bone – the osteoporosis connection revisited. Proc Soc Exp Biol Med 219:1–7

www.ingramcontent.com/pod-product-compliance
Lightning Source LLC
Chambersburg PA
CBHW051829170526
45167CB00005B/2219